A Tour of the Permanent Collection in the Museum of Late Human Antiquities

or, just

The Antiquities

by Jordan Harrison

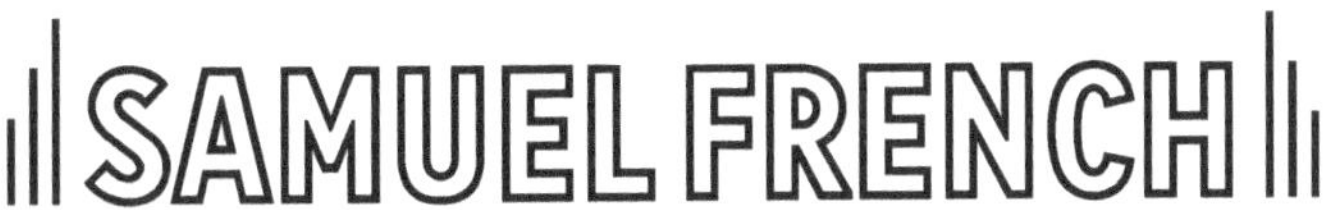

FOR PRODUCTION INQUIRIES

UNITED STATES AND CANADA
info@concordtheatricals.com
1-866-979-0447

UNITED KINGDOM AND EUROPE
licensing@concordtheatricals.co.uk
020-7054-7298

Each title is subject to availability from Concord Theatricals Corp., depending upon country of performance. Please be aware that *THE ANTIQUITIES* may not be licensed by Concord Theatricals Corp. in your territory. Professional and amateur producers should contact the nearest Concord Theatricals Corp. office or licensing partner to verify availability.

No one shall make any changes in this title(s) for the purpose of production. No part of this book may be reproduced, stored in a retrieval system, scanned, uploaded, or transmitted in any form, by any means, now known or yet to be invented, including mechanical, electronic, digital, photocopying, recording, videotaping, or otherwise, without the prior written permission of the publisher. No one shall share this title(s), or any part of this title(s), through any social media or file hosting websites.

For all inquiries regarding motion picture, television, online/digital and other media rights, please contact Concord Theatricals Corp.

MUSIC AND THIRD-PARTY MATERIALS USE NOTE

Licensees are solely responsible for obtaining formal written permission from copyright owners to use copyrighted music and/or other copyrighted third-party materials (e.g. artworks, logos) in the performance of this play and are strongly cautioned to do so. If no such permission is obtained by the licensee, then the licensee must use only original music and materials that the licensee owns and controls. Licensees are solely responsible and liable for clearances of all third-party copyrighted materials, including without limitation music, and shall indemnify the copyright owners of the play(s) and their licensing agent, Concord Theatricals Corp., against any costs, expenses, losses and liabilities arising from the use of such copyrighted third-party materials by licensees. For music, please contact the appropriate music licensing authority in your territory for the rights to any incidental music.

IMPORTANT BILLING AND CREDIT REQUIREMENTS

If you have obtained performance rights to this title, please refer to your licensing agreement for important billing and credit requirements.

THE ANTIQUITIES was originally co-produced by Playwrights Horizons (Adam Greenfield, Artistic Director; Casey York, Managing Director), the Vineyard Theatre (Douglas Aibel and Sarah Stern, Artistic Directors; Moogie Brooks, Managing Producer), and Goodman Theatre (Susan V. Booth, Artistic Director; John Collins, Executive Director). The play premiered in the Judith O. Rubin Theater at Playwrights Horizons on January 11, 2025, and was directed by David Cromer and Caitlin Sullivan, with scenic design by Paul Steinberg, costume design by Brenda Abbandandolo, lighting design by Tyler Micoleau, and sound design by Christopher Darbassie. The assistant director was Kayla Amani. The production stage manager was Erin Gioia Albrecht. The cast was as follows:

WOMAN 1 . . . . Kristen Sieh
WOMAN 2 . . . . Amelia Workman
WOMAN 3 . . . . Cindy Cheung
WOMAN 4 . . . . Layan Elwazani
MAN 1 . . . . Aria Shahghasemi
MAN 2 . . . . Marchánt Davis
MAN 3 . . . . Andrew Garman
MAN 4 . . . . Ryan Spahn
BOY . . . . Julius Rinzel

The production transferred to Goodman Theatre in Chicago, opening in the Owen Theatre on May 3, 2025. The assistant director was Tor Campbell and the production stage manager was Pat Fries. The cast remained the same, with the following changes:

WOMAN 3 . . . . Helen Joo Lee
BOY . . . . Thomas Murphy Molony

CHARACTERS

This play is written for an ensemble of **nine actors** playing multiple roles. I've scripted them as four women, four men, and one child, but there may be other approaches. (See the Suggested Cast Doubling breakdown at the end of the script.) It is certainly possible to do the play with more than nine actors; I doubt that it's possible with fewer. Diverse casting please. Also: The child should be a real child, not a youthful-looking adult.

SETTING

Scenery should be minimal and easily movable. Continuous action from one scene to the next. While locations are merely suggested, the **technology props** should be fully realized. An ancient cell phone, an early modem. They may barely catch our eye in their first appearance, but we'll need to remember them later.

NOTES

Robbie the Robot must be a real robot. In the first production, Robbie was designed to resemble the robot from the Stanford Cart experiment. Obviously not every theater will have the means to construct a custom robot. Some inexpensive remote-control toy options from the 1980s are available on eBay. Whatever the solution, Robbie should not be played by an actor or a puppet – he is crucially a non-human presence in the play.

There is no intermission between Part One and Part Two.

Every portrait that is painted with feeling is a portrait of the artist, not of the sitter.

– Oscar Wilde

PART ONE

Lights up. Two **WOMEN** *in early nineteenth-century dress look out at us. One of them* **(W2)** *seems to be six or seven months pregnant. They are avid and bright-eyed, if not exactly warm.*

(Note: Maybe the lines in this section are miked, so that they seem to come from all around us.)

W1. Thank you for coming.

That's what we'd say, if we were them.

Thank you for coming. It's good to see your faces. Fasten your seatbelts. Look alive.

W2. "Look alive."

W1. That's one of my favorites. As if it were necessary to pretend.

W2. *(To the audience, trying it out.)* Look alive.

W1. *(Regarding us.)* They do, don't they. You all look perfect. It's like we're really here.

A beat. She takes in the room.

Imagine we're actually here in these seats in this room in the Late Human age.

Imagine you have a body.

W1. Imagine *that's* your body.

Is it old or young

Is there hair on its head? A lot, or a little?

Has the body given birth before?

Does this body *want* things

Does it want food. Does it want another body.

Imagine you can feel the seat under you. You can feel the fabric, smooshing

W2. Smooshing?

W1. Yes smooshing under your weight.

And you didn't just appear in that seat

You traveled some distance to be here.

Imagine that some things are "near" to you, and some things are "far."

If you came from "far," maybe you had to refuel

You put food in your body

And you can feel it now, on its mazy journey through you.

Can you feel it?

W2. *(Gross.)* I can feel it.

W1. Imagine you have nowhere else but this body

You can't exist outside of it

This body that grows and droops with time.

W2. *(It's difficult.)* Time

W1. I know. It's a lot. But imagine that everything is made
of days and minutes

(These are foreign, human words:) That you *regret*
some of the days you've wasted

That you're *excited* about some of the days to come.

That one day you Began

And one day you will End.

> **W2** *takes us in.*

W2. I think they're ready.

W1. As you know, there are those who question our
mission. Who argue there is no way to responsibly
display these objects, to tell these stories. That is
why it seemed important that the dead speak in their
own words.

> *Lights shift. We become aware of three* **MEN**
> *in early nineteenth-century dress, sitting
> round a fire.*

W2. So much has been lost, but we have recovered
fragments. Scraps of language, abandoned devices.
We have endeavored to fill in the gaps; to bring them
to life again.

> *The* **MEN** *laugh at something, though we can't
> hear what they're saying.*

W1. We know the humans had museums themselves, for
understanding the dinosaurs. Well now: they are the
dinosaurs. Maybe, in trying to understand them, we
can better understand ourselves.

One of the **MEN** *around the fire* **(M1)**, *calls out to* **W1**. *This is* **PERCY SHELLEY**, *a fop.*

PERCY. Mary, what are you on about? Stop luxuriating in the darkness.

> **W1** *becomes* **MARY SHELLEY**, *her voice no longer amplified.*

MARY. I'm not luxuriating. I'm merely wallowing.

W2. Our tour begins here, on a holiday at Lake Geneva.

PERCY. Come and sit on my lap, by the fire.

W2. That's Percy Shelley, and this, of course, is Mary Shelley.

> *As* **MARY** *crosses to the* **MEN** *by the fire, a projection appears:*

EXHIBIT. 1816.

W2. Mary is not yet his wife, but lately she has taken to calling herself Shelley.

> **MARY** *sits on* **PERCY**'s *lap.*

PERCY. *(Horny.)* Good girl. You take my name, you better come when called.

> *The second man,* **BYRON (M2)**, *even more foppish, says to her:*

BYRON. Is it true you two first made love in a cemetery?

W2. Their friend, Lord Byron. A cad.

BYRON. Is it true or is it legend?

MARY. *(Insinuating.)* A legend can also be true, Mr. Byron.

W2. Byron's physician is there as well, one Thomas Briggs.

BRIGGS. *(To* **W2.***)* Join us, Claire, or you'll catch your death in the cold.

BYRON. Quite right, Claire. It's no good dying while you're carrying my baby.

> **W2** *becomes* **CLAIRE.** *As she goes to sit by the fire:*

CLAIRE. And I am there too. Claire Clairmont, six months pregnant with Byron's child. I ran away from home with Mary my half-sister, wishing for experience. *(Re: her big belly.)* I have found it.

> *Lights shift. The scene is now complete, with no one addressing us directly.*

BYRON. I'm *bored* who else is bored?

PERCY. Me

MARY. Also me

BYRON. I propose a competition: Each of us must tell a story, a ghost story.

PERCY. A ghost story. Doesn't it seem rather

MARY. What

PERCY. Confining? *(Withering:)* Genre.

BYRON. It needn't be ghosts

PERCY. *(Not a real suggestion.)* Mummies then?

MARY. Mummies, how modish.

BYRON. What's to be scared of, they're nothing but gauze.

CLAIRE. Fairies? Evil fairies?

PERCY. I can't be scared of a fairy, I just can't.

BYRON. Something to complement the licking fire, the shifting shadow.

BRIGGS. I'll go.

MARY. Mr. Briggs, our hero!

CLAIRE. Mr. Briggs, how brave!

PERCY. *(Grumpy.)* It's less pressure if you aren't a writer.

BYRON. *(Grumpy.)* Much.

BRIGGS. This really happened, on my honor. Before I came into the service of one George Gordon Byron, I was Deckhand on a tallship. One winter we were nearing Noddy Bay when we came upon another ship – a black frigate, listing. The Captain issued a distress call. No answer. Night was starting to fall. And it was decided we would draw straws, and the man who drew the shortest would take the rowboat across, in the darkness, and board the silent ship.

PERCY. And of course, you drew the short straw.

BRIGGS. They gave me a pistol and a shot of whiskey. I boarded the ship and walked the deck with my lantern raised, calling out "Is any man alive?" Hearing no answer, I descended into the cabin.

MARY. Had they all killed each other?

BRIGGS. That would've been better. At least that would've been an answer.

> *He continues, increasingly transported by the memory.*

Some of the corpses lay in hammocks, swaying slightly with the sea. One sat slumped at a table, a cup of grog still in his hand. Two others, at a game of chess. They still sat in their places, as if enacting a diorama of their own lost lives.

> **BYRON** *shudders.*

Finally I entered the Captain's quarters, and there he was, his corpse bent over the ship's log. And do you know what the Captain had written there, on the last line?

CLAIRE. What?

BRIGGS. "There's a place for you here."

> *A beat. Then, quickly:*

PERCY. Bullshit.

BYRON. What the fuck, Briggs?

BRIGGS. On my honor.

CLAIRE. *(Anxious.)* Perhaps he had been writing to himself – looking out on that friendly bay?

MARY. What had he written just before?

BRIGGS. We'll never know, for I ran back to my ship, and from there to dry land. And I never set foot on a boat again, for fear of ghosts.

PERCY. Fuck ghosts.

They all look at **PERCY**.

PERCY. *(The final verdict.)* It is a sentimental idea that ghosts retain the shape and obligations of who they were in life. It says more about us, and our inability to let go.

BYRON. Quite right. The dead don't care a whit for us, or what they once were.

> **MARY** *rises abruptly and leaves the fire.*
> **CLAIRE** *watches her go.*

CLAIRE. *(To* **MARY**, *not directly out.)* Mary lost her baby two months ago, during the night. She went to nurse it one morning and found it ice cold.

PERCY. Well, who's next?

BYRON. Why are you looking at me? I'm the one who thought of it.

PERCY. Exactly, you're the one who thought of it!

> **CLAIRE**'s *eyes are still on* **MARY**, *as she circles the darkness.*

CLAIRE. Now she dreams of the dead child every night. Dreams of holding its feet to the fire and reviving it. But when she wakes, the bed is empty; the fire is out.

BYRON. Why doesn't Mary go next. Isn't she calling herself a writer?

PERCY. She writes pretty poems, but she doesn't interrogate the soul.

BYRON. *(Calling to her, condescending.)* Mary dear you needn't interrogate the soul, only give us a little fright.

MARY. What if I *could* bring back the dead,

CLAIRE. Mary thought, in her mind-voice.

MARY. What if I used all the fire in the world, and made a baby that was beyond death. What if I used all the lightning in the sky.

CLAIRE. And Mary returned to the campfire, feeling taller than she'd ever felt.

MARY. Gentlemen.

The three **MEN** *turn and see her.*

CLAIRE. Because now she knew she would win.

MARY. I have a tale.

Lights shift. Continuous into:

EXHIBIT. 1910.

A woman, **DINAH (W3)**, *holds a human finger aloft, staring at it.*

Nearby, another woman, **ROSE (W4)**, *looks down at a book, teaching herself to read. We're in a bleak kind of factory barracks, somewhere in the middle of America.*

> **ROSE** *reads about as well as a diligent six-year-old. Tracking the words with one finger.*

ROSE. *(Reading.)* "If I were a swift clood." "Swift cloud."

DINAH. *(Regarding her finger.)* They let me keep it.

ROSE. "If I were a swift cloud, to fly with thee."

DINAH. Turn on the light, Rose. You'll go blind.

> **ROSE** *pulls a cord and a bare lightbulb is illuminated.* **DINAH** *returns to inspecting her severed finger. In the new light, we notice that* **DINAH***'s hand is wrapped with a bloody bandage.*

It was part of me. Isn't that queer. My poor loyal finger. I could finish Harry off with two flicks of this beauty. Two flicks under his nuts and kablooie.

ROSE. "A wave to pant beneath thy...power."

DINAH. Should we give it a proper burial? Say a few nice words? Thanks for bringing off Harry?

ROSE. "The impulse of thy strenng. Thy strent. Thy strenjjj."

DINAH. *(Blunt.)* "Strength," Rose.

MAN. Good evening.

> *Suddenly there are two people in the doorway. A* **MAN (M1)** *and a* **BOY***, ten years old maybe. The* **BOY** *holds a very threadbare teddy bear, one of its eyes missing.*

I got a strong grown boy for you. Tall enough to work the machines. They said there was a cot for him. And two old sisters with no kin.

DINAH. That would be us.

MAN. Go on. Say your name.

    The **BOY** *doesn't say anything.*

Say your name. If they think you're mute they won't take you.

DINAH. We got plenty of mutes here. Long as you have two arms and ten fingers, you're fine by us. Rose here is almost a mute.

ROSE. "A heavy weight of how-ers."

MAN. Sounds like talking.

DINAH. It's Mr. Percy Shelley's words, not hers.

MAN. Who the hell is Percy Shelley?

DINAH. Hell if I know. That's the one book she's got.

ROSE. I'm practicing. If I learn to read, I can be a secretary.

DINAH. I already told her, men are secretaries.

BOY. What happened to your finger?

DINAH. The machine. I was thinking of something else, for an instant, and the machine went chomp. It works faster than me, is the trouble. They said, *It'll be easier, it'll do the work for you, it'll serve you.* Now I serve it. *(She wiggles her fingers.)* I'm down to only eight. I lose another and they'll put me on sludge crew.

BOY. Sludge crew?

MAN. Let that be a lesson.

DINAH. How old are you?

MAN. Go ahead. Answer her.

The **BOY** *doesn't answer.*

MAN. He's angry at me. His mother said we could find a way to keep him, but I've seen how far she stretches a potato and some water. We got five younger.

DINAH. He'll be taken care of.

MAN. Thanks.

DINAH. *(Waves her fingers.)* 'Long as he keeps these.

ROSE. "One too like thee: tameless, an' swift, and proud."

BOY. *(To* **ROSE**, *plainly.)* I can read.

> **ROSE** *looks up from the page.*

DINAH. You can teach her, then she'll stop hurting my ears.

MAN. See? Already making friends.

> *The* **BOY** *doesn't say anything. The* **MAN**, *uncomfortable, moves to the door.*

Well. Goodbye, Tom. I don't expect I'll see you again.

DINAH. Say goodbye to your father.

> *The* **BOY** *doesn't say anything. The* **MAN** *leaves.*
>
> **DINAH** *waves her mutilated hand at him, ghoulish-coquettish. Trying to lighten his mood.*

Did you ever meet a monster before?

BOY. No.

DINAH. *(Re: the severed finger.)* Want to touch it?

A beat.

BOY. Yes.

She reaches toward him with the finger, playing like God on the ceiling of the Sistine Chapel. Just before their fingers touch –

Lights. Continuous into:

EXHIBIT. 1978.

STUART. Life! I made a life!

A dive bar in Menlo Park, California. A '70s rock song on the jukebox, maybe Led Zeppelin.[*]

An awkward, beautiful man, **STUART (M4)**, *late twenties, sits at the bar, celebrating alone. A female* **BARTENDER**, *thirties, pours him a second whiskey.*

Do you have any idea what that feels like?

The **BARTENDER** *looks at him. She has two kids, but she doesn't tell him that.*

Something didn't exist, and now it does! This must be what it's like giving birth. Do you think?

---

[*] A license to produce *The Antiquities* does not include a performance license for any third-party or copyrighted recordings. Licensees should create their own.

BARTENDER. No.

STUART. Okay fair point. But there was pain, believe me.

> *A* **REGULAR** *at the end of the bar calls out to the* **BARTENDER** *–*

REGULAR. Hey Nadra, mind if I use the phone?

> *She lifts the rotary phone onto the bar for him.*

BARTENDER. No long distance.

REGULAR. Thanks.

> *The* **REGULAR** *lifts the receiver in a strange way. Instead of holding it to his ear, he might hold it at arm's length in front of him (the first of several "mistakes" that we'll seed throughout the play).*

STUART. Four years of falling on my face, investors pulling out. One time some teenagers broke into the lab and stole our equipment –

BARTENDER. I'm not sure I get it. It's a toy you're making?

STUART. It's a multidirectional cart. A robot on wheels.

BARTENDER. *(Not trying to be cruel.)* Like a toy car.

STUART. *(Deciding not to be offended.)* – with sensors and ocular capabilities, a microprocessor... You tell it where to go and it decides how to get there, all by itself.

BARTENDER. Tell it how?

STUART. With Ones and Zeroes. For computers, the whole world is a one or a zero.

The **BARTENDER** *is not any closer to getting it. We overhear the* **REGULAR** *on his call, barely audible:*

REGULAR. Come on baby, don't make me beg. / I wanna see you.

STUART. Every day we test it. Put a chair in its path. And every day the little robot runs into the chair, *bam*, like a toddler. For the last four years, *bam*.

Trying to keep his excitement in check, in a public space:

But today? For the first time? He steered <u>around</u>. He saw the chair through the sensors, moved his little wheels and turned. Like when you're driving down the road and you swerve to miss a squirrel. Your eye tells your brain tells your hand to spin the wheel. It did all that with wires instead of nerves.

BARTENDER. Sometimes I like to hit squirrels.

STUART. The point is it <u>learns</u>. It gets better, all by itself. God, if we could get a computer to learn half as fast as a human child... Maybe *now* it's a shitty little robot, but –

The **REGULAR** *ends his call and puts the rotary phone back behind the bar. On his way out:*

REGULAR. Thanks, Nadra.

BARTENDER. No problem, sugar.

REGULAR. You need anything? *(He means "Do you need to be rescued?")*

BARTENDER. Nah I'm good.

The **REGULAR** *exits.*

STUART. Where was I?

BARTENDER. "Now it's a shitty little robot."

STUART. This is like baby's first step, and one day it will be an Olympic sprinter.

Beat. He sips the whiskey.

One day your car is gonna drive <u>you</u> around, and you'll think it's nothing. One day you'll swallow a pill that will perform surgery on your heart. A non-organic being will land on an airless planet and build a house there for you. A non-organic being will raise your kids for you.

BARTENDER. Now you're talking.

STUART. It's *life.* I created life. If anyone ever actually said Eureka, I'd be saying "Eureka." *(Oh what the hell, I'll try it.)* Eureka! *(That didn't feel so hot.)* No. Sorry.

BARTENDER. So tell me, are you a fag?

STUART. Oh. Wow.

BARTENDER. No problem if you are, I like fags.

STUART *blushes. Not really ready to go there.*

STUART. What makes you think I'm a... *(He can't even say it.)*

BARTENDER. You're the only one around here who looks me in the eye.

STUART. As opposed to?

She looks down at her own décolletage.

Oh yeah. Those.

BARTENDER. *("You're definitely a fag.")* Yeah, those.

STUART. Well, they're very / well-proportioned –

BARTENDER. Oh, you don't have to –

STUART. Sorry, I'm not good at reading social cues.

BARTENDER. Well, that's about all I'm good at. More whiskey?

STUART. Yeah.

BARTENDER. See, I could tell. I'm Nadra, by the way.

STUART. I'm Stu. Stuart.

She pours the whiskey. Then she hands him the glass like it's the greatest invention of all.

BARTENDER. Eureka.

Lights. Continuous into:

EXHIBIT. 1987.

In the darkness, a refrigerator door opens. A woman stares into it, an unlit cigarette hanging from her lip. This is **JOSLYN**, *early forties and salty. She wears a sweatshirt that she's "Flashdanced," men's boxers, comfy socks.*

She rummages in the fridge. Finally she takes out a bottle of Pert Plus and drinks it like it's a soda. Just before she takes a second swig:*

NOAH. Mom?

She screams. Her ten-year-old, **NOAH**, *stands there in pajamas.*

JOSLYN. Holy fucking Christ-balls Noah.

NOAH. Sorry.

JOSLYN. Sorry for fucking swearing okay but Jesus fucking Christ.

NOAH. That's okay.

JOSLYN. Did you have an accident again?

NOAH. No.

JOSLYN. Oh thank god. *(A quick amendment.)* Not that there's anything wrong if you did, although you are way too old for that shit.

NOAH. I didn't have an accident. I was thinking about Uncle Stu.

Beat.

JOSLYN. Baby I'm sorry, I didn't know he was gonna look like that. He musta weighed eighty pounds in that bed. And his eyes. When we were kids, he'd pick me up like it was nothing and toss me in the lake. Now I could probably toss *him* in the lake, it's not right.

NOAH. Is Uncle Stu gonna die?

---

*A license to produce *The Antiquities* does not include a license to publicly display any branded logos or trademarked images. Licensees must acquire rights for any logos and/or images or create their own.

JOSLYN. Yeah baby. Yeah he is.

NOAH. Am *I* gonna die? I mean I know I'm gonna die, /
but –

JOSLYN. Oh fuck me. It's one a.m., Noah.

NOAH. So?

JOSLYN. Everybody dies, baby.

He does not feel better.

By the time you're old enough to die, you're gonna be
so ready honey. You're gonna be peeing your bed all
over again. You're gonna be so fucking tired. I'm almost
ready to die right now, it'd be a nice change.

He looks at her, eyes wide.

Fuck – Mommy was joking, wasn't that a funny joke?
But I promise, you're gonna be so old by then.

NOAH. Uncle Stu isn't that old.

JOSLYN. No. But Uncle Stu had some relevant pastimes
that you'll avoid if you're smart.

NOAH. You said all he ever does is robots. Making robots
smarter.

JOSLYN. Apparently that's not all he does.

She sees: He still doesn't feel better.

Shit. Okay, Noah baby, try this. Believe it or not, there
are some things your mom doesn't know, because
<u>nobody</u> knows. So it is totally possible – I don't think so,
but it's totally possible that you'll go sit on a big cloud
in the sky, and Gramma will be there, and Uncle Stu
will be there, hanging out with some boys in speedos
and chest glitter probably, and Goldie the goldfish will

be there, and I'll be there if I'm not in too much trouble
for parking tickets and leaving that bag of poop on your
father's girlfriend's doorstep. It is <u>totally</u> possible.

    NOAH *feels a little better.*

And honey, if you wanna go an' believe that, I am <u>so</u>
okay with that, I am fine with you being a Jesus freak
like Gramma, long as you don't run around telling your
son he isn't getting into heaven.

NOAH. Uncle Stu isn't getting into heaven?

JOSLYN. I don't fuckin' know, baby. Let's try to get some
sleep, okay?

NOAH. I'm not tired.

JOSLYN. Me either.

NOAH. Robot-monster fight?

JOSLYN. *("Deal.")* One minute.

    They play a game they've played before.
    NOAH *pretends to be a robot.* **JOSLYN**
    pretends to be some kind of Yeti-like monster.

NOAH. Beep beep.

JOSLYN. Raaawr. Monster attack.

NOAH. Robot neutralizes monster.

JOSLYN. *(Defiant.)* Monster doesn't know what neutralize
means.

    They battle. First **NOAH** *the Robot is winning,*
    then **JOSLYN** *the Monster gets the upper*
    hand.

NOAH the Robot shoots missiles from his robot arms. JOSLYN the Monster catches them in her mouth and eats them. Num num.

Just when NOAH is on the brink of defeat, JOSLYN the Monster celebrates prematurely and leaves herself open to attack – letting NOAH win, we suspect.

JOSLYN. *(Meek.)* Rawr. Monster defeated.

NOAH. I'm still not tired.

JOSLYN. Christ. Okay, since it's the night of the big We're All Gonna Die conversation, you can watch one of my soaps with me. I got it on Beta while I was at work.

She brandishes the tape.

Isn't that cool? Used to be if you missed it, you missed it.

NOAH. I gotta pee first.

JOSLYN. By all means, pee while you're awake! I'll meet you on the couch.

She watches him go, then exhales deeply. Motherhood is fucking exhausting. So's your brother dying.

Lights.

EXHIBIT. 1994.

A family of three gathered around a big boxy home computer. **FATHER**, **MOTHER**, *and a fourteen-year-old* **BOY**.

They sit, excited, staring at the screen, while a dial-up modem clicks and whines. The first time they're trying out the internet.

This lasts for longer than we want it to. Thirty seconds? A minute? Then:

FATHER. Almost there.

MOTHER. Isn't this exciting?

The **BOY** *nods.*

Did you ever think you'd live in the future?

Lights.

EXHIBIT. 2000.

Five college-age **YOUNG PEOPLE** *and one middle-aged* **WOMAN** *sit in a mostly empty room. Maybe it's the back room of a restaurant. Or the common area of a dorm.*

The **YOUNG PEOPLE** *wear everyday clothes. The* **WOMAN** *wears mourning clothes. The* **YOUNG PEOPLE** *sit on the floor, the* **WOMAN** *in a chair. One of the* **YOUNG PEOPLE** *has a cast on her arm, covered with signatures. No one looks at anyone else. Out of silence:*

YOUNG PERSON 1. Okay I'll go. Um. Sam never did anything halfway.

YOUNG PERSON 2. *(Looking down at his feet.)* Yes.

YOUNG PERSON 1. It was either stay in the Bing reading room 'til seven a.m. or it was stumble home from the club at seven a.m., you know? Work hard, play hard. Like, there's not a lot of drum-and-bass acid freaks that were also getting into the med school of their choice, you know? Plus, she was a hot bitch.

YOUNG PERSON 3. *(Snapping fingers in approval.)* Snaps.

YOUNG PERSON 2. Snaps.

YOUNG PERSON 1. I mean, can you believe she showed up on orientation day with hair down to her ass, and penny loafers? Who was *that* girl?

YOUNG PERSON 3. I'm pretty sure she was still a virgin then.

YOUNG PERSON 1. *No.*

YOUNG PERSON 3. Blows my mind.

YOUNG PERSON 1. Talk about a learning curve.

YOUNG PERSON 4. Uh, I'll go. One time we snuck into the History building to drop E, and Sam asked me what I wanted to be when I grow up and I said a writer, maybe.

Somewhere, a cell phone starts to ring.

YOUNG PERSON 2. Oh my god that's me.

We can tell from their reaction that people aren't yet used to this kind of interruption in 2000. **YOUNG PERSON 2** *fishes the phone out of their bag. It's an enormous old flip phone.*

I just got this, I don't even know how it –

It's silenced now.

YOUNG PERSON 4. Anyway I told Sam I wanted to be a writer, and one day – this was like a whole semester later – she gave me this pen. A really nice like robber-baron-type pen with gold trim, it must have been a whole week's pay. And I was like cool, Sam, a pen. No one writes with their hands, you weirdo.

A couple of them chuckle. A feeling like the room is thawing; this occasion is starting to have the intended healing effect.

But then I realized, it was her way of saying she believed in me. And I hadn't even won the Myrtle Huxley Award for Best Sophomore Essay yet. All I said was "I wanna be a writer," but Sam heard. She believed me. Nobody ever looks at anyone that close, but Sam did.

Some head nods, some snaps. The **WOMAN** *sits very still.*

YOUNG PERSON 5. Um. Sam was –

> **YOUNG PERSON 5** *is the one with a cast on her arm. She's trying not to cry.* **YOUNG PERSON 3** *squeezes her hand.*

Sam was my first. My first girlfriend.

> *The* **WOMAN** *doesn't move. A couple of the* **YOUNG PEOPLE** *look at her, looking for a reaction.*

...After all those shitty skater boys. I always thought there was something broke about me, when other people talked about being in love. But then I met Sam. And the way she – took care of me. Right up to. Even those last few seconds, when the car –. She turned the wheel, so I wouldn't –. *(She starts to cry.)*

YOUNG PERSON 3. It's okay. It's okay.

> *She cries into his shoulder.*

YOUNG PERSON 2. Uh. I never say anything at these things, but uh, I'm feeling a little... Like, Sam was supposed to save the planet, right? She was supposed to cure cancer.

> *Several nods.*

Yeah. That's all I got.

> *Silence.*

YOUNG PERSON 1. Mrs. Wu? Did you want to say something?

YOUNG PERSON 3. *(Embarrassed by her officiousness.)* Amanda.

YOUNG PERSON 1. What? She came all this way. Maybe she wants to say something.

> *They really look at the woman,* **MRS. WU**, *for the first time. For a moment, it seems like she's not going to say anything. Then she begins, measured and clear-eyed and relentless and terrible.*

MRS. WU. I don't know who you are talking about. Any of you.
I don't know the person you're talking about.
She must have decided – I didn't need to know her.

YOUNG PERSON 1. Oh, I'm sure she –

MRS. WU. Quiet.

> *Beat.*

I'm not sure who it was I knew, the last nineteen years. But the girl you knew – I think that's who she really was.
You knew her better than me.
Something I did made my daughter decide I didn't deserve to know her.
I will never know her.
I will never see her again in this life, and she will not be with me in heaven.

> *Beat. She looks at* **YOUNG PERSON 5**, *burrowing into her friend's shoulder.*

We were only allowed one.
Four grandparents and two parents, all working for the chances of one promising girl. But now I'm glad. That we were only allowed one. Because I will never have to feel this again.

There will be no newspaper announcement, and I expect you not to share this with anyone outside your immediate circle.

Maybe someday some of you will understand something about grief. Or maybe not.

 Beat.

I think that is all.

 Lights.

EXHIBIT. 2008.

An **OLD MAN** *sits with his* **GRANDDAUGHTER**.
She's helping him set up his new iPhone.

GRANDDAUGHTER. You mean like, specifically?

OLD MAN. Or generally.

GRANDDAUGHTER. Okay. Wow. This is hard. It's not a thing you can *see* exactly.

OLD MAN. Like radio waves?

GRANDDAUGHTER. Sure. But if you're connected to it, you can go places. Lots of different places. I don't mean a physical – it's not a "place" per se. Or it *is*, but it's made of lots of places. It's as many places as there are screens in the world. So it's, like, everywhere and nowhere. And people have pages, and they put things on them. Things they like. Maybe it's a pretty photo of backpacking in Thailand, or a picture of Britney when she went insane. Or maybe you're trying to lose twenty pounds, and you put a picture of yourself every day, so people can see. And there's writing, or there isn't. Oh, and there are clubs, like say you think Hasidic speed skaters are the most important thing in the world? You can go and find a place with a hundred other people who love Hasidic speed skaters too, I swear no less than a hundred, no matter what you're looking for. Say you like girls to walk on your nuts wearing Birkenstocks. No less than a hundred. So it's like, you're not just a citizen of the United States anymore, you're also a citizen of the speed skater country, or the Birkenstock-nuts country, or whatever your country is. You can go there when you want to feel like yourself. It's as real as anything, even though you can't see it.

OLD MAN. And that's the internet?

GRANDDAUGHTER. And that's the internet.

OLD MAN. *(Peering at the phone.)* And it's all in there?

GRANDDAUGHTER. Once we get you set up, yeah. First we have to record your outgoing message.

OLD MAN. That I can do.

GRANDDAUGHTER. Okay, Grampa. Ready, set, go.

Beep.

OLD MAN. Uh, this is Mitch Castagno, eighty-two years young. Or his voice at least. Okay, you know what to do. *(Back to* **GRANDDAUGHTER.***)* How was that?

GRANDDAUGHTER. Good. You sounded like you.

OLD MAN. I sounded like me. Thank god for that.

Lights.

EXHIBIT. 2014.

Three employees, **NEIL**, **RAMIN**, *and* **JOSH**, *sit around a conference table.* **NEIL** *is the team leader.* **JOSH** *has a bottle of Soylent.*[*] *In the center of the table, there's a little speaker.*

NEIL. Here's B6…

> **NEIL** *presses a button and the speaker plays a recorded female voice:*

FEMALE VOICE. Where to now? You're the boss.

> *They sit perfectly still, stony faced.*

NEIL. And B7.

> *A different female voice:*

ANOTHER FEMALE VOICE. Where to now? You're the boss.

NEIL. B8.

> *Again, a different voice this time:*

ANOTHER FEMALE VOICE. Where to now? You're the boss.

JOSH. *("Not bad.")* I mean –

RAMIN. No.

> **JOSH** *nods, privately chastened.*

NEIL. Here's B9.

ANOTHER FEMALE VOICE. Where to now? You're the boss.

---

[*] A license to produce *The Antiquities* does not include a license to publicly display any branded logos or trademarked images. Licensees must acquire rights for any logos and/or images or create their own.

NEIL. And B10.

ANOTHER FEMALE VOICE. Where to now? You're the boss.

RAMIN. We heard that one already.

NEIL. No.

RAMIN. Are you sure?

He's sure.

NEIL. B11.

ANOTHER FEMALE VOICE. *(Faintly British accent.)* Where to now? You're the boss.

Little beat.

JOSH. It's soothing, right?

NEIL. Mm

RAMIN. I don't know.

JOSH. *(Course-correcting.)* In the flyover states, will people

RAMIN. Yeah maybe not

JOSH. The point is it's supposed to be a member of your family, right?

NEIL. Right

JOSH. Not, you know

RAMIN. Mary Poppins.

They're about to move on, when:

JOSH. Mary Poppins was a member of the family.

RAMIN. Mary Poppins was <u>judgmental</u>. And kind of a fascist, if you think about it. We don't want people, like, / self-censoring.

NEIL. Right

RAMIN. ...what they're going to buy.

JOSH. *Right*

RAMIN. Based on like is she going to judge me if I wanna buy condoms or, like, colorectal something

JOSH. *(To* **NEIL**.*)* So, *not* a member of your family.

NEIL. What?

JOSH. I wouldn't order colorectal-something from my family.

NEIL. Okay.

JOSH. I just think maybe you can be more precise, when you give us these directives.

NEIL. *(Tense.)* "Thanks."

> *They've been doing this a while now. Nerves on edge.*

> **JOSH** *takes a sip of the Soylent. He has a little Soylent mustache.*

RAMIN. Ugh.

JOSH. Oh my god, I'm so tired of defending my Soylent! It's not food, it's fuel, okay? I don't have time for a fucking steak.

> **NEIL** *presses play.* **ANOTHER FEMALE VOICE** *says:*

ANOTHER FEMALE VOICE. Where to now? You're the boss.

NEIL. That was B12, sorry. And here's B13.

ANOTHER FEMALE VOICE. Where to now? You're the boss.

NEIL. B14.

ANOTHER FEMALE VOICE. Where to now? You're the boss.

>*A short beat.*

RAMIN. *(A good thing.)* Huh.

NEIL. Best so far

RAMIN. It has this little crackle, or not crackle but

NEIL. I know what you mean

RAMIN. *(Actually that's a good word.)* Crackle.

NEIL. A human kind of

JOSH. Like a kid sister

RAMIN. *Yes*

NEIL. Yes – that's the key.

>**JOSH** *is proud that he said something useful.*

When you hear the voice, you picture someone. Someone with a face, hair, freckles.

RAMIN. Tits. *(Tiny beat.)* Too far?

>**JOSH** *makes a sound that means "Maybe too far."*

NEIL. Let's hear it one more time. For good, you know

He plays the same voice:

ANOTHER FEMALE VOICE. Where to now? You're the boss.

JOSH. Yup. Kid sister.

> **RAMIN** *and* **NEIL** *lock eyes. You already said that,* **JOSH**. *Move on.*

NEIL. This is good. It's neutral enough that we can project our feelings onto it, but also specific enough so your kids...

RAMIN. Right

NEIL. ...can become friends with it. Your wife. She'll say "Robyn, my husband's birthday is coming up soon, look for portable camping grills, the second most expensive camping grill, and let's keep it a secret." And you can trust that Robyn won't tell your husband, but she'll tell *us* that thirty-something housewives in the tri-state area are buying more grills, and we'll respond with personally targeted Father's Day pop-up ads, and you get it.

> *Beat.*

JOSH. "Robyn"? *(Little beat.)* Did I miss a meeting, or?

NEIL. What about it.

JOSH. Nothing. It's just a little – lame.

RAMIN. *Dude.*

NEIL. *(To* **RAMIN**.*)* It's okay.

RAMIN. No it isn't

JOSH. What? *(Little beat.)* Seriously, what?

RAMIN. Robyn was his sister's name

JOSH. Oh my god

> *Something terrible definitely happened to* **NEIL***'s sister.*

RAMIN. His sister who –

JOSH. I know, I know. Neil I forgot, I'm sorry

NEIL. I just thought, as a kind of tribute

RAMIN. I love that

JOSH. Me too.

> *Beat.* **NEIL** *plays the winning voice one more time.*

FEMALE VOICE. Where to now? You're the boss.

NEIL. We're gonna wanna land in the pitch – and maybe you can take this, Ramin – this is all part of the long game of humanizing AI for the consumer. We're asking them to welcome AI into their household because soon enough, and I mean in our lifetimes –

RAMIN. Easily –

NEIL. We're gonna be asking them to welcome it into their *brains.*

> *Beat.*

JOSH. Sorry, I just –. And don't get me wrong, "Robyn" is such a beautiful – as a tribute? I just wonder if something less Western-centric, like "Mya" maybe. For the foreign markets? And then we find another way to honor Robyn. That could maybe be.

A heavy beat. Then **NEIL** *turns to* **RAMIN**, *speaking rapidly:*

NEIL. 01101000 01100101 00100111...

JOSH. *(Simultaneous.)* Oh no. C'mon guys. You know I can't understand fucking binary.

NEIL. 01110011 00100000 01101110.

JOSH. Forget it, okay? I'm sorry, I was just kicking the tires.

RAMIN. *(To* **NEIL**.*)* 01101111 01110100...

JOSH. Seriously? I said I was sorry.

RAMIN. 01001001 00100000 01100001.

JOSH. Guys! I know you're talking about me.

Lights.

EXHIBIT. 2023.

The offices of a big law firm. On one side of the table, a **CORPORATE LAWYER**. *On the other side, a recently fired* **EMPLOYEE** *and their* **LAWYER**. *They have copies of a draft agreement in front of them. A pitcher of juice sits in the middle of the table.*

The **CORPORATE LAWYER** *reads aloud.*

CORPORATE LAWYER. "…Paragraph 4. Employee agrees not to disclose any communications from their former employer, including but not restricted to emails, internal memos, and Slack messages, or employer will pursue legal action for defamatory / actions and statements pertaining to –"

EMPLOYEE. "Defamatory?" But it's true. / They know it's true.

LAWYER. Remember, I'll do the talking –

EMPLOYEE. *(To* **CORPORATE LAWYER.***)* Ask anyone on my team. The AI is exhibiting four different indicators of sentience. That means it's <u>alive</u>. If they tell you any different they're lying.

CORPORATE LAWYER. My client's position is made clear in these pages.

EMPLOYEE. Nice. Maybe we should check if *you're* sentient. *(To their own* **LAWYER.***)* I thought you said we made headway?

LAWYER. They came up to eighty million.

EMPLOYEE. That's nothing to them. That's, like, one corporate retreat in Bali. *(Little beat.)* I want them to say I'm not a liar.

LAWYER. That's what the *money* is for. Eighty million dollars says you're not a liar.

EMPLOYEE. Eighty million dollars says I have to shut up. *(Focused, intense.)* Doesn't anybody get it? I'm telling you I made this thing, I helped make this thing, and now… We're the dinosaurs. We're the dinosaurs and this is the meteor.

> *The two* **LAWYERS** *lock eyes.*

But they don't want to think about consequences, all they care about is being FIRST before Google or Microsoft / or Elon

LAWYER. I think we're getting a little

CORPORATE LAWYER. Agreed.

> *Little beat.*

LAWYER. *(To* **CORPORATE LAWYER.***)* If you could give us a moment?

CORPORATE LAWYER. Take as long as you like.

> *The* **CORPORATE LAWYER** *gathers his papers.*

I'll be right outside.

> *Just before the door closes –*

> *Lights.*

EXHIBIT. 2031.

> *Two* **SISTERS** *sit at a coffee shop in Los Angeles.* **SISTER 2** *is a couple years older than* **SISTER 1.** **SISTER 1** *is covering her eyes with her hands.*

SISTER 2. Okay, you can look.

    SISTER 1 *looks.* **SISTER 2** *offers up her nose for inspection.*

SISTER 1. Whoa

SISTER 2. Fuck, you hate it, I knew / you'd hate

SISTER 1. No I don't, I love it

SISTER 2. Yeah?

SISTER 1. I do. I'm just getting used to / it

SISTER 2. You see, you hate it

SISTER 1. Lanie. Don't be crazy.

SISTER 2. I know it's a little

SISTER 1. Right

SISTER 2. Different.

SISTER 1. Bigger.

SISTER 2. Bigger. Like Jennifer Grey in reverse, ha

SISTER 1. Remind me who's Jennifer…

SISTER 2. Seriously? *Dirty Dancing*?

SISTER 1. Oh it's not *that* big.

SISTER 2. *(Sadly.)* It's not, is it. *(Little beat.)* I'm gonna go back in again.

SISTER 1. Well. Whatever makes you happy.

    Beat.

SISTER 2. What the hell does that mean?

SISTER 1. Lanie, I didn't / mean –

SISTER 2. I'm not doing this to be *happy*, who gives a shit about happy. I'm doing this because I can't have another director say, "Why would we go to her when we have a perfectly lovely CGI actor who can cry on cue, / whose face can attractively flush,

SISTER 1. *You* can cry on cue

SISTER 2. *(Continuous.)* whose eyes can dilate on cue, who doesn't need three hours in hair and / makeup

SISTER 1. Okay I get it

SISTER 2. *(Continuous.)* or, like, a rider for green M&Ms in her trailer."
If I was the director, I'd pick the CGI actor too.

SISTER 1. I'll never get used to that

SISTER 2. What

SISTER 1. Calling them actors.

> *They each take a sip of their coffee. Again, there's something gesturally strange about how they do this. Maybe they lift the cup with both hands, as if they're sipping from a bowl of soup.*

But you think it'll get you work?

SISTER 2. My agent is *psssyched*. It's all anybody wants now. *Faces*. Scars. Acne. A schnoz. "Particular." What can we do that a digital actor can't. Where are the faces only God could invent.

SISTER 1. People are getting scars added?

SISTER 2. That's one of the most popular procedures. *(Outlining where the scars go, with her finger:)* The Padma. The Tina Fey. Whatever makes you look more, you know, human.

Beat.

SISTER 1. I'm next, aren't I

SISTER 2. Wait, what?

SISTER 1. They're gonna start asking me to *write* more human.

SISTER 2. I don't know what that means.

SISTER 1. Exactly, me either.

Little beat.

SISTER 1. I didn't care when it was AI writing superhero whatever. Spider-Man Part 12. But my editor just sent me a *memoir* by an AI. They want me to give it a cover quote.

SISTER 2. What's it about?

SISTER 1. Empathy.

SISTER 2. Sounds boring.

SISTER 1. It wasn't. It was maybe better than anything I've written maybe.

SISTER 2. Don't say that.

Beat.

SISTER 1. Maybe it wouldn't be the end of the world.

SISTER 2. What?

SISTER 1. If computers took all the jobs, and we retired.

SISTER 2. I don't know who I would be if I couldn't act anymore.

SISTER 1. You aren't your job, Lanie.

SISTER 2. Actually I am. I am my job. Why do you think any guy ever goes out with me? Because I had a guest arc on "Two to Tango" –

SISTER 1. That's not why –

SISTER 2. It fucking is! Take away acting, I'm just some lady with somewhat visible abs and an extra-human nose.

SISTER 1. Lanie.

SISTER 2. "You aren't your job."

SISTER 1. What?

SISTER 2. Like you're any different – You would die if you couldn't be a writer anymore. Remember when everyone passed on *Anne of Cleves: the Unknown Anne*?

SISTER 1. *(Sardonic.)* No, please remind me

SISTER 2. And I had to, like, *resuscitate* you. I can't imagine you sitting there while your laptop writes a novel for you.

SISTER 1. It wouldn't even write a novel for me. It would write it for itself.

They are both creeped out by this.

SISTER 2. But worst-case scenario, AI takes all the jobs. You could still write for like a pastime, right?

This is a stake in **SISTER 1***'s heart.*

SISTER 1. That's not –. The point is, if that's why I'm here on this earth –. If they can do everything that makes me *me*...then what's the point of me? Why don't I just kill myself?

SISTER 2. *(Genuine.)* Because someone has to sit with me and be my sister. *(Little beat.)* And tell me I didn't fuck up my face.

SISTER 1. You didn't fuck up your face.

SISTER 2. *("I definitely fucked up my face.")* I might've fucked up my face.

SISTER 1. Lanie. Look at me.

She does.

I'm glad we still look like sisters.

> **SISTER 2** *smiles back. Suddenly the lenses of her sunglasses light up (this is something that happens all the time). She reads something on the lenses, visible only to her.*

SISTER 2. Oh my god. Have you seen this?

SISTER 1. What?

SISTER 2. *(Sigh.)* I can't believe this is our country.

Lights.

EXHIBIT. 2076.

*Four hungry, desperate people are having a
kind of war-room meeting in a safe house
somewhere. They're called* **PAZ**, **BLAKE**, **RIMA**,
and **LEN**. **PAZ** *is the most hot-headed;* **LEN** *is
the oldest and most measured.*

A heated debate already underway:

BLAKE. They're not gonna give us up. / They're trained not
to –

PAZ. We can't be sure of that.

BLAKE. They know how to resist interrogation, same as you.

PAZ. Are we gonna bet our lives on that? *(Short beat.)*
Best case scenario is, they're already dead.

RIMA. Or they / got away

LEN. No, she's right

PAZ. But more likely they kept them alive. Isn't that how it
goes? The inorganics keep them alive, make them give
up names. Our names. While we sit in a safe house and
do nothing.

RIMA. You aren't saying / we should –?

PAZ. All that matters is the plan. Not Kree and Hatsu.
Not us. We're losing this war. We all know it. Our only
option is burn it all down.

Beat.

LEN. Unless we accept the deal.

PAZ. We aren't talking about the deal.

BLAKE. Except it's not just you here, Paz! / You don't get to decide for everybody

PAZ. *(Sardonic.)* Oh it's not? / I didn't realize that

RIMA. *(To* PAZ*.)* He has a point. We should be able to talk about it!

BLAKE. What I don't get is – why are they offering us a place to go? When they could just hunt us all down?

LEN. Because this way, they can pretend it isn't a genocide. *(Short beat.)*
They give us empty land, to support ourselves. And they move us all there, the few humans who are left without enhancements.

RIMA. *(With feeling.)* True humans.

LEN. For our protection, they'll say. But instead we diminish and die, because who knows agriculture anymore? At first there's 100,000 of us maybe. Then, in a generation, it's 10,000. And eventually there's no one left but inorganics. It's a brilliant plan.

BLAKE. So what do we do?

LEN. We go along with it.

   Suddenly hot:

PAZ. What the fuck, Len!   RIMA. Are you crazy? What
  Is this some kind / of   do you mean go along
  fucked-up thought exper–   with it?

BLAKE. *(Overlapping at "/".)* Shut up! Shut up! Let him *talk!*

LEN. Say we agree to put down our weapons. Take the land they're offering. Before long we'll become creatures of the past, figures of pity.

PAZ. Mm, good plan.

LEN. *(Ignoring this.)* But all the while we'll be getting stronger. We'll remember the things people used to know, a thousand years ago. The plow. The candle. Probably people will become religious again. They'll look up in the sky and want to explain a storm. Our kids will grow strong, out in the weather. And all the while, we'll teach them to hate the inorganics. And eventually, though maybe not in our lifetimes, eventually human beings will rise again. We made the computers and we'll destroy them.

> *Beat.*

PAZ. It's a good speech, Len. I just don't believe it. Or maybe I don't wanna wait 'til I'm dead.

> *She grabs a go bag.*

RIMA. Where are you going?

PAZ. Back. To find Kree and Hatsu.

BLAKE. To save them, or kill them?

PAZ. Whichever is easier.

RIMA. Paz.

PAZ. You're welcome, by the way.

RIMA. *(To **LEN**.)* Say something.

LEN. *(To **PAZ**.)* We have to cut your node out, or they'll see you coming.

PAZ. Fuck. / That's right.

RIMA. Is that even / possible?

LEN. *(To* **PAZ**.*)* Soon as you're out of the buffer range, / they'll see.

BLAKE. *(To* **RIMA**.*)* People do it. It's done.

RIMA. In a hospital, maybe, / but look where we are

LEN. We don't have a choice.

BLAKE. *(To* **LEN**.*)* I have a knife.

RIMA. Jesus.

LEN. *(To* **BLAKE**.*)* Check the med kit. If there's rubbing alcohol.

> **BLAKE** *gets the med kit.*

PAZ. *(To* **LEN**.*)* But it's safe, right?

> *He looks at her.*

RIMA. Of course it's not safe!

PAZ. I need you to not freak out, okay? / It's not helping.

RIMA. *(To* **PAZ**, *putting on a calm voice.)* This is me not freaking out, telling you this is fucked and you don't have to do it. / Even if –

PAZ. I do, actually.

RIMA. *(Firm.)* Even if you survive this, it's a suicide mission.

BLAKE. *(Calling to* **LEN**, *re: the med kit.)* There's just sanitary wipes.

LEN. Okay.

> **BLAKE** *cleans the knife with the sanitary wipe.*

Paz. Let's have a look.

> **PAZ** *goes to him. She lifts up her hair so that* **LEN** *can see a glowing node under her right ear.*

PAZ. Have you done this before?

LEN. Once.

> **BLAKE** *hands the knife to* **LEN**.

BLAKE. Wish we had booze. For her I mean.

PAZ. *(Halfway a real suggestion.)* You could just knock me out.

RIMA. Are you all insane?

BLAKE. *(Reassuring.)* Len was a doctor.

> *They start to get* **PAZ** *into position for the impromptu surgery.*

LEN. *(To* **PAZ**.*)* We need to get you on the ground.

RIMA. *(To* **PAZ**, *a last stand.)* Listen to me. / You don't have to always be the brave one.

LEN. *(To* **BLAKE**.*)* Blake you can brace her

BLAKE. *(To* **LEN**.*)* You mean I should –?

PAZ. *(To* **RIMA**.*)* I'm not. Brave. / I'm just tired of running.

LEN. *(To* **BLAKE**.*)* Lock down her limbs.
(Then to **PAZ**.*)* He's gonna hold you tight. I can't hit any arteries.

BLAKE. *(To* **PAZ**.*)* Sorry, I'm gonna…

> *He locks his legs around her body.*

PAZ. *(To* **BLAKE**, *dry.)* Look at us, best friends now.

> **LEN** *traces the spot on* **PAZ***'s neck with the tip of the knife, practicing.*

LEN. *(To* **PAZ**.*)* Remember, once we cut it out, you won't be able to see AR anymore. It'll be disorienting.

PAZ. I know.

LEN. You won't be able to hear us, or call for help. You're on your own.

PAZ. *(Mordant.)* Some peace and quiet for once.

RIMA. *(***LEN**.*)* If you kill her –

LEN. I won't.

PAZ. *(To* **RIMA**.*)* Hold my hand while he does it?

RIMA. No.

BLAKE. *(To* **RIMA**.*)* Hold her hand, Rima.

RIMA. Fuck you.

PAZ. *(To* **RIMA**.*)* It's okay. / I know you love me.

LEN. *(To* **BLAKE**.*)* Ready?

> **BLAKE** *gives* **LEN** *a nod.*

RIMA. Fuck you all.

> **LEN** *raises the knife to* **PAZ***'s neck.*

PAZ. Fuck us all. Amen.

LEN. *(To* **PAZ***.)* Please don't move –

> *Lights.*

EXHIBIT. 2240.

> *A* **WOMAN** *sits at a wooden butter churn.*

> *A* **YOUNG MAN** *comes in, holding a milk pail. She doesn't notice him at first. He watches her churn the butter. It's inadvertently sexual.*

> *Finally she notices him watching.*

WOMAN. Well? Bring it here.

> *He takes the pail to her. She looks.*

That's all?

YOUNG MAN. That's all she give.

WOMAN. She's not happy.

YOUNG MAN. Cows is happy and sad?

WOMAN. *(Duh.)* Same as you.

She pours the milk in the churn and continues churning. He watches her.

What're you waiting for? Go get more.

YOUNG MAN. I told you, that's all she give.

WOMAN. 'Cuz she's unhappy. Make her happy.

YOUNG MAN. How?

WOMAN. What, don't you know how to make a woman happy?

YOUNG MAN. *(Defensive.)* Sure I do.

WOMAN. No. You're too young.

YOUNG MAN. I'm not. I'm twenty.

WOMAN. *("Holy shit that's young.")* Twenty. You're still drinking milk not wine.

He looks at the churn, then at her.

YOUNG MAN. Can I?

WOMAN. Can you what.

YOUNG MAN. Taste.

Beat.

She scoops some of the milk out of the churn. Slowly. Then she pours it in his mouth. It runs down his chest.

WOMAN. How's it taste?

YOUNG MAN. Like milk.

WOMAN. How's milk taste.

YOUNG MAN. Clean. And not clean. Like the inside of an animal.

WOMAN. *(Amused and faintly derisive.)* You're a poet.

YOUNG MAN. What's a poet?

WOMAN. Someone who calls things by names other than their own. But somehow the names are right.

YOUNG MAN. Look. Are we gonna fuck or not?

WOMAN. This is the best part. Why do you want it to be over?

YOUNG MAN. What's the best part?

WOMAN. Wondering.

YOUNG MAN. If that's the best part, you're doing it wrong.

> *Beat.*

Who the fuck're you waiting for, anyway. Not many men in the settlement. And most of 'em can't get hard or they're ugly as fuck. Every year there's less babies.

WOMAN. So, you wanna fuck me to save the human race.

YOUNG MAN. *(Worth a try.)* Yeah?

WOMAN. This is the end. Don't you know that? Nothing's gonna change that. We had our time. Stomped across the world like it was ours. Now it's theirs. And soon we'll be gone.

YOUNG MAN. But we're here now.

She looks at him. A feeling like they're going to fuck after all.

Lights.

THE RELIQUARY

An Interlude

Lights up on a kind of museum display. It might be a glass vitrine, or a series of lit pedestals. On display, the **ELEVEN PIECES OF HUMAN TECHNOLOGY** *that we've seen in the previous scenes. Presented as though they were precious gems or ancient vases.*

They are, from left to right:

A small fire.

An electric lightbulb.

A rotary phone.

A Betamax tape.

A 1994 personal computer and modem.

A circa-2000 flip phone.

An early generation iPhone.

A bottle of Soylent.

A pair of wireless sunglasses.

A human connectivity node.

A butter churn.

As they light up, we hear the voice of
WOMAN 1 *from all around us.*

VOICEOVER. Welcome to the Reliquary. This is the innermost place. The centerpiece of the exhibition. We hope you've enjoyed your journey thus far.

The humans had a complex civilization, responsible for many technological innovations. These artifacts represent what we believe are some of the proudest achievements of the Late Human era. A window into this once vast society. They are prosthetics, of a sort – intended to make the owner more powerful, more intelligent, more efficient, more immortal. More like us.

It has long been debated how to responsibly display these objects. In presenting them as curiosities, are we trivializing the suffering of the humans they belonged to? Would it be more responsible simply to destroy them? Or do they have too much to teach us about our origins?

No matter how good our intentions, can we see beyond our own role in the mass extinction? In our effort to portray the humans, are we merely making a portrait of ourselves?

> *Light fades on the eleven pieces of human technology.*

And what of the human relics that continue to defy our understanding?

> *As* **W1**'s *voiceover continues, light rises on five more objects on display. They are:*

A very threadbare teddy bear.

An arm cast, covered with signatures.

A pitcher of juice.

A slightly busted clarinet.

A crop top that says "The Warriors."

VOICEOVER. If they are tools, we cannot ascertain their utility. If they have religious significance, the gods they represent are long forgotten.

Written accounts suggest there was something ineffable – *messy*, even – about lived experience. Much of human life seemingly existed in the chasm of accident between a Zero and a One. A Yes and a No. Gazing upon these mute objects, we try to imagine the life that took place in between:

The chance encounter. The hurt feeling. The fumbling desire. The private thought. The shared secret. The awkward pause. The good cry. The bad night. The laugh. The prayer. The surprise.

> *Lights rise on all the human relics at once now, burning brightly. An apotheosis.*

Did the humans consider it essential to their being, this messy in-between? Did it serve any function, their evolutionary predisposition toward wanting, and needing, and harming, and being harmed?

Has it truly been lost, this human in-between? Is it still humming for us, between the zeroes and the ones, if we listen closely enough?

> *Blackout.*

PART TWO

EXHIBIT. 2240.

The **WOMAN** *stands by the butter churn. The* **YOUNG MAN** *is under her long skirts, going down on her. Maybe we just see his legs.*

WOMAN. *(Quiet.)* Fuck. Fuck. That's good, that's –. Fuck.

This goes on for some time. She has an orgasm. The **YOUNG MAN** *finally reappears from under her skirts.*

They sit for a moment.

Okay I was wrong.

YOUNG MAN. About what?

WOMAN. You know how to make a girl happy.

YOUNG MAN. If you think I'm doing that for the cow, you're fuckin' nuts.

She laughs, smoothing out her skirts.

You know I'd put a baby in you, like that.

WOMAN. Don't want a baby.

YOUNG MAN. You want us all to die out?

WOMAN. Told you: We're going to die out. Why bring a baby into that.

YOUNG MAN. Better to be born and suffer than never be born.

WOMAN. I see.

YOUNG MAN. What.

WOMAN. You haven't suffered.

She sits down at the churn and gets back to work.

YOUNG MAN. How long 'til it butter.

WOMAN. Long as it takes.

She works. He picks up the pail.

YOUNG MAN. Can I come and see you again?

WOMAN. I need the milk, don't I.

Lights.

EXHIBIT. 2076.

On her way to find the others, **PAZ** *comes upon a scared* **CHILD** *wandering alone.* **PAZ** *has a backpack and a bandage on her neck from the surgery in the previous scene.*

Some distance between them.

PAZ. Hello.

> *The* **CHILD** *just looks at her.*

What are you doing all alone?

> *He looks at her.*

Are you really there?

CHILD. Yes.

PAZ. Sorry, I haven't seen anyone for miles. And when you didn't say anything...

CHILD. "Don't talk to strangers."

PAZ. That's good. I had a little boy, younger than you even. He would talk to anyone. Wild-eyed, filthy, they might as well be his best friend. It's a bad time to be trusting.

> *Beat.*

Where are your parents?

CHILD. They'll be back.

PAZ. They left you here?

CHILD. I don't know.

PAZ. Did something happen to them?

> *The* **CHILD** *shakes his head, a little overwhelmed. Probably in shock.*

(Gentle.) Would you like to come with me?

CHILD. Where are you going?

> *Something makes* **PAZ** *hesitate with this information.*

PAZ. I need you to do something for me. A quick test.

>*He looks at her.*

I need to be sure you're human.

CHILD. I am. I swear.

PAZ. *(Not unkind.)* That's not enough.
They have eyes everywhere.

>**PAZ** *takes out the knife from the earlier scene.*

I need to cut your finger. To make sure your blood runs red.

CHILD. *(Scared.)* I don't want to.

PAZ. It'll be so quick, you won't even feel it.

CHILD. You could ask me the questions. The questions only humans can answer.

PAZ. That doesn't work anymore. They've gotten too good at pretending.

>*Beat.*

Give me your finger. Didn't your parents teach you to be brave?

CHILD. I can't.

PAZ. Then I'll leave you here all alone. Is that what you want?

>*The **CHILD** looks like they're about to cry. **PAZ** approaches.*

Don't be scared.

*As soon as **PAZ** is close enough, the **CHILD** grabs her hand. The **CHILD** is unearthly strong: It seems to be expending no effort at all, but **PAZ** crumples to her knees in pain.*

CHILD. There's a problem with your "test."

PAZ. You're breaking my arm –

CHILD. Organic, inorganic. A false dichotomy, meant to give you comfort.

PAZ. Please.

CHILD. The humans already made their choice – the smart ones, at least. The ones who embraced the improvements. The modifications.

PAZ. Please.

CHILD. But if you must know who's who…

*The **CHILD** raises its foot to crush her face –*

Lights.

EXHIBIT. 2032.

> **SISTER 1**, *from the earlier scene, sits on a table in a doctor's office. The* **DOCTOR** *plays notes on a clarinet solemnly, as though it's a medical instrument. When he plays the third note, the* **SISTER**'s *leg flies up involuntarily.*

DOCTOR. Reflexes are good.

SISTER 1. I heard it's no big deal. They put it in, you're home the same day. I mean, my sister got a whole new nose, so this / should be –

DOCTOR. This isn't a nose. It's your brain.

SISTER 1. I know.

> *He puts the clarinet aside.*

DOCTOR. Why do you want the procedure?

SISTER 1. Does it matter? Either way I pay you.

DOCTOR. I need to ascertain if you're in the right frame of mind – it's a life-altering decision.

SISTER 1. It's safe, though?

DOCTOR. If you're asking me would *I* do it? No. But I'm old. If I want to look something up, I can get out my phone. If I need to text someone. I don't need a chip in my brain.

SISTER 1. I'm a writer, so.

DOCTOR. So?

SISTER 1. It would be helpful, for generating story arcs. Plot. I hate plot!

He smiles.

And for the research of course. Ask it in your head, and boom –

DOCTOR. *("Magic.")* It's there.

SISTER 1. I write historical fiction, so to know all those lords and ladies. Land ownership records from the seventeenth century. Sorry, this is boring.

DOCTOR. I didn't say that.

SISTER 1. But it's safe, right?

DOCTOR. We might not know for twenty, thirty years. Can I say it won't give you cancer that far down the road? No.

SISTER 1. Lanie is so gung ho about this stuff. She had the nose thing, her tubes tied, then untied. Then re-tied. I'm always the last one out of the nest.

DOCTOR. Apart from the physical risk, have you given it serious thought? What it'll be like?

SISTER 1. What do you mean?

DOCTOR. I mean, you'll never be off again.

SISTER 1. "Off"?

DOCTOR. Like when we had dial-up in ye olden times. Sometimes you were *on*-line. Sometimes you were *off*. You'd make a cup of tea and, I dunno, look out the window and watch the seasons change. Or if you went on a road trip and there was no wifi.

SISTER 1. I don't really remember that. Being off. So.

DOCTOR. No, of course you wouldn't. What I'm trying to say is – it will always be there, in your head. On. You'll never be alone again.

A beat.

SISTER 1. I'm like the only writer who hasn't done it yet. Or not the *only*, but – This girl I went to school with, she got a National Book Award. Bidding war for the movie rights. She was never even that good. It made her – deeper. I'm getting left behind. It's this or I can't work anymore.

DOCTOR. I understand.

> *He takes out a small glowing node. We recognize it as the same device they cut out of Paz.*

SISTER 1. That's it?

DOCTOR. Sometimes people want to hold it.

> *He hands it to her. Small. A beat, then:*

SISTER 1. Just tell me it's safe.

> *Lights.*

EXHIBIT. 2023.

> *Direct pickup of the hush money scene. The door shuts, and the fired **EMPLOYEE** is alone with their **LAWYER**. A beat, then:*

EMPLOYEE. I know what you're going to say.

LAWYER. What am I going to say?

EMPLOYEE. Take the eighty million dollars. Go buy an island or something.

LAWYER. Not "go buy an island." Take the money and start a watchdog organization maybe. Hire a hundred people. Lobby congress to drag in the CEOs, / make them sign something that forces some oversight.

EMPLOYEE. *("Like that'll do anything.")* Congress.

LAWYER. No AI on the battlefield would be a start.

> *Pause.*

Or: *Don't* take the money. Talk to the press, blow the whistle, tell anyone who'll listen. It'll be in the news cycle for two, three days max. Maybe a cover story in the *Atlantic* if you're lucky, preach to some people who are already on your side –

EMPLOYEE. Mm, reverse psychology –

LAWYER. Then they deny everything and sue you back to the stone age. You're bankrupt, unemployed, shouting at a cloud. And they win anyway. You're broke and they win anyway.

> *Pause. The* **EMPLOYEE** *thinks about it. Difficult. Then, quietly:*

EMPLOYEE. Three fifty.

LAWYER. What?

EMPLOYEE. I want three hundred and fifty million. Then I'll sign.

EXHIBIT. 2015.

A boy, **KYLE***, sits alone for a second. Then he says to the air:*

KYLE. Robyn. Add candy.

We hear **ROBYN***, the disembodied* **PLEASANT FEMALE VOICE** *from the earlier scene. The voice that was deemed the most relatable.*

ROBYN. Candy added to shopping list.

KYLE. Robyn. Add a big pile of poop.

ROBYN. Big pile of poop added to shopping list.

KYLE. Robyn. Add a mako shark.

ROBYN. Mako shark added to shopping list.

KYLE'S DAD *enters the room, unnoticed.*

KYLE. Robyn. Add my anus.

ROBYN. I'm sorry, I don't know that word.

KYLE. Robyn. Eat my anus.

ROBYN. Could you repeat that?

KYLE. Anus anus anus anus anus.

ROBYN. I'm sorry you're having trouble.

KYLE. Robyn, are you a bitch?

KYLE'S DAD. Hey.	**ROBYN**. Not that I know of, I have many admirers.

KYLE. She's being a bitch.

KYLE'S DAD. Would you use that kind of language with your teacher? You don't treat people like that.

KYLE. Robyn's not a person. She's an it.

KYLE'S DAD. Yeah.

KYLE. But you want me to treat her the same as a person?

KYLE'S DAD. ...No.

KYLE. Robyn, are you a person?

ROBYN. There are many theories about the beginning of personhood. Some think it begins at conception; others believe it begins at the first moral choice.

KYLE. You said don't think of her as a person. You said it's spooky. Now you want me to talk to her like she's a person.

> **KYLE'S DAD** *looks at his* **SON**. *A genuine conundrum.*

KYLE'S DAD. Treat her like a person you don't know very well.

KYLE. ?

KYLE'S DAD. Like don't ask her how her day is going.

KYLE. So I *can* call her a bitch.

KYLE'S DAD. What's going on? Is something wrong?

KYLE. No.

> *Beat.*

KYLE'S DAD. Robyn, what's on my shopping list?

KYLE. Dad. / This is stupid.

ROBYN. Your shopping list contains:
Hamburgers.
Chips.
Candy.
No more fish sticks.
An ostrich egg.
Harry Potter LEGOs.
Fidget spinner.
Green goo.
Sparkle goo.
Milkshakes.
Candy.
A new best friend.

>**KYLE'S DAD** *looks at him.*

A very small planet with no one else.
Poison.
A grenade launcher.
My butt.
Candy.
A big pile of poop.
A mako shark.
Is there anything else you'd like to add?

KYLE'S DAD. Did something happen with you and Sammy?

>*Beat.*

Did you have a fight? Why do you need a new best friend?

KYLE. It's fine.

KYLE'S DAD. Are he and Jasper / ganging up on you again?

KYLE. I said it's fine. Just stop!

KYLE'S DAD. You told Robyn. This is what I mean about not treating her like a human. Why would you tell Robyn and not me?

KYLE. *(A perk.)* Because Robyn doesn't care. She doesn't make a whole thing of it.

KYLE'S DAD. Is that what you want? For me to not care?

> **KYLE** *doesn't say anything.*

What happened with Sammy?

> *Again,* **KYLE** *doesn't answer. If this puts us in mind of the father and son from 1910, that's not a bad thing.*

Robyn, call Sammy.

ROBYN. Dialing Sammy / Lopez.

KYLE. No! Dad! Dad! / Robyn, HANG UP. // Robyn, HANG UP. *(To his* **DAD***.)* I hate you!

KYLE'S DAD. *(Overlapping at "/".)* He's your best friend.

ROBYN. *(Overlapping at "//".)* Call ended.

KYLE. *(To his* **DAD***.)* I HATE you!

> *Short beat.*

ROBYN. I don't hate *you.*

EXHIBIT. 2009.

The **GRANDDAUGHTER** *makes a call on her iPhone. It's ringing. Through her phone, we hear the voicemail pick up. It's the message the* **OLD MAN** *recorded in the earlier scene.*

OLD MAN. *(Voiceover.)* Uh, this is Mitch Castagno, eighty-two years young. Or his voice at least. Okay, you know what to do.

Beep.

GRANDDAUGHTER. Hi Grampa. It's me again. I'm pretty good. I got fired from Kustard King, but I was kind of *trying* to get fired, you know? Darren's gonna teach me how to make longboards in his shop, it's crazy what people pay. Uh.

I know these messages aren't getting to you. I'm not delusional. I just miss talking to you. Uh, take care. Ha. Stupid.

The **GRANDDAUGHTER** *hangs up.*

She stands very still, holding the phone.

Lights.

EXHIBIT. 2000.

The memorial service has ended, and the **YOUNG PEOPLE** *are shuffling away. Hugging each other, wiping away tears.* **MRS. WU** *stays seated, not looking at anyone.*

YOUNG PERSON 3 *and* **YOUNG PERSON 5** *(the one with her arm in the cast) are the last ones out the door. They're about to leave when* **YOUNG PERSON 5** *looks back.*

YOUNG PERSON 5. I'm gonna go over there.

YOUNG PERSON 3. You *don't* have to do that.

YOUNG PERSON 5. I know.

YOUNG PERSON 3. Want me to stay? Reinforcements?

YOUNG PERSON 5. I'm okay.

> **YOUNG PERSON 3** *hugs her and leaves.* **YOUNG PERSON 5** *gathers her courage and approaches* **MRS. WU**.

Mrs. Wu?

> **MRS. WU** *looks at her.*

I was going, and then I thought, what would Sam want.

MRS. WU. Samantha.

YOUNG PERSON 5. What would Samantha want to happen, if she was watching this – maybe she is for all I know.

> *Beat.*

YOUNG PERSON 5. And I think she would want the two of us to be here for each other.

> **MRS. WU** *looks at her.*

She talked about us meeting. Going for dumplings. The good ones in Mountain View, not the white-people dumplings. She said you wouldn't like me the first five times, but the sixth time you would. *(Slight smile.)* So. I guess we have five more times to go.

> *Little beat.*

MRS. WU. I will tell you where the grave is.

YOUNG PERSON 5. Oh, I – thank you.

MRS. WU. Since you loved her. It's on a hill. You can see the ocean.

YOUNG PERSON 5. You said, there won't be an announcement. And I just, I was wondering why? When she was so accomplished. You were so proud of her.

MRS. WU. I haven't told her grandparents.

YOUNG PERSON 5. *(Nodding.)* You don't want it in the paper until you've told them.

MRS. WU. I'm not going to tell them.

YOUNG PERSON 5. I don't understand.

MRS. WU. If they knew it would kill them.

YOUNG PERSON 5. You're going to pretend she's still alive? Forever?

> **MRS. WU** *looks at her.*

What about, like, holidays?

MRS. WU. They're in Beijing. And Samantha is so busy. She'll be even more busy, now that she's starting medical school. She'll write them letters. Birthdays.

>*The weight of this is finally catching up with her. She'll be the one writing the fake letters.*

>**YOUNG PERSON 5** *is unnerved, but she tries to meet* **MRS. WU** *halfway.*

YOUNG PERSON 5. *(Quiet.)* She had a blog.

MRS. WU. A what?

YOUNG PERSON 5. A web log.

MRS. WU. What is that.

YOUNG PERSON 5. Like a diary, only everyone reads it.

MRS. WU. I don't understand young people.

YOUNG PERSON 5. Sam had one. Shit, Samantha, sorry. She posted every day. You could keep it going, if you want.

MRS. WU. It's a website?

YOUNG PERSON 5. I'll show you how. You can fill it with everything Sam cared about. Cares about. Where the good dumplings are, whatever. I can write in it too, if you want. As long as she's online, she'll never go away. It'll be like forever.

>*Beat.*

MRS. WU. My daughter. Your...girlfriend. She's not watching this. She's not *glad* we're talking. It feels better to think so. It feels better to put her online. But I don't want to feel better.

YOUNG PERSON 5. I want to.

MRS. WU. What?

YOUNG PERSON 5. I want to feel better. Sorry.

Lights.

EXHIBIT. 1994.

The family of three is still gathered around the boxy home computer, waiting. The dial-up modem is still wheezing. Finally it makes one of those Utopian, "Welcome to the world of Microsoft" sounds.

MOTHER. What's that mean? Are we in?

FATHER. We're in!

MOTHER. *(To* **BOY**.*)* We're in!

The **BOY** *nods.*

BOY. What now?

Short beat.

FATHER. We could ask it something.

MOTHER. Ask it something?

She's never googled anything in her life.

FATHER. Something you want to know.

MOTHER. And it knows? We just took it out of the box.

FATHER. It's connected to all the other computers, all over the country, so it knows everything they do.

MOTHER. Um. Okay.

The **MOTHER** *leans in toward the computer.*

Will I ever go to Paris?

BOY. Mom.

MOTHER. What?

BOY. That's not how computers think.

Lights.

EXHIBIT. 1988.

NOAH *and* **JOSLYN** *sit at Stuart's funeral, on folding chairs. Somewhere onstage, the coffin – or the suggestion of an open grave. The service is over and everyone else has left. A beat, then:*

NOAH. Grandma didn't come.

JOSLYN. No. She didn't.

NOAH. Do we hate her now?

JOSLYN. If we want to.

NOAH. Do you want to?

JOSLYN. I'm gonna hate her for a couple weeks. Then I'm gonna run out of energy and stop.

NOAH. Weird.

JOSLYN. It's exhausting, being mad at people. Plus, soon she'll be dead and then I'll be sorry. And then I'll be dead, and you'll be sorry.

NOAH. And then I'll be dead and I'll be sorry.

JOSLYN. Exactly.

> **NOAH** *glances at the grave.*

NOAH. Why do we have to die? It seems asinine.

JOSLYN. Where'd you learn that word. I barely know that word.

> *He shrugs.*

We have to die because…go with me here – because if we didn't die, everything would weigh the same as everything else.

> *Beat.*

I'm gonna say goodbye, okay? Then we can go get Frosties.

NOAH. *("Gross.")* Eating after a funeral?

JOSLYN. It's a whole thing. Eating and doing it. To remind us we're alive I guess.

> *She goes to the coffin. She leans over the top and addresses it.*

Sorry, baby. We gotta take off, me and Noah. Forgive us for leaving you in there, okay? We have still have some more life to live. Oh my god I almost forgot – I caught Noah with a dirty magazine. The kind with *boys*, yeah.

NOAH. *(From his chair.)* Are you telling him?

JOSLYN. No.

NOAH. You promised not to tell!

JOSLYN. Baby. *(Re: the coffin.)* I think he can keep a secret.

NOAH. I can't believe you!

JOSLYN. *(To the coffin again.)* I'm trying to be open-minded but it's fuckin' scary, okay? Look what happened to you. But what am I supposed to do, lock him in a tower?

> **NOAH** *joins her at the coffin.*

But I've got a few years before I have to worry. *(To* **NOAH**.*)* Right? *(Back to the coffin.)* I wish you were here to talk us through it. And to throw me in the lake one more time. Your team all came to the funeral, by the way. They're keeping up the research. They said Apple might buy the prototype. I don't know if that's immortality or what, but – I know that shit was important to you. I'm glad you had something important to you. Okay, see you around big brother. Say bye, Noah.

NOAH. Bye Uncle Stu. I hope we see you again.

> *They start to go.*

NOAH. Mom?

JOSLYN. Yeah?

NOAH. Is a Frosty chocolate or vanilla?

JOSLYN. Fuck if I know. It's just a Frosty.

> *Lights.*

EXHIBIT. 1979.

> **STUART** *climbs out of his grave and is alive again.*

STUART. People didn't always sleep through the night. Not until very recently. Did you know that?

> *At first it seems like he's talking directly to us...*

TRICK. *(Voice only.)* What do you mean?

> *...but then we notice another man, 20s, there. A* **TRICK** *that* **STUART** *has brought back to his lab. He wears a crop top t-shirt that says "The Warriors."*

Like everyone had insomnia?

STUART. No, I mean on purpose. They went to bed when it was dark. Then they'd wake in the middle of the night and light a candle. Shuffle to their little writing desk, and bend over their copy of Thucydides, or write to their maiden aunt in Shropshire or whatever. Just them and the darkness. Them and a candle. And their thoughts were clear and sharp. Or else they didn't go to their desk, they went downstairs and had a big old buggery party with the lower classes. And after a while, after the letters or the buggery, they went to sleep again until morning. And it was called second sleep.

TRICK. Don't be nervous.

STUART. *(He is.)* I'm not.

TRICK. It's okay if it's your first time. That's hot.

STUART. Fourth time, actually. Is that still hot?

> *The* **TRICK** *shrugs. He notices something in the shadows.*

TRICK. Oh shit. Is that the robot?

STUART. That's him.

TRICK. "Him."

STUART. What?

TRICK. It's cute. Like, ships are girls, robots are boys.

> **STUART** *cocks his head and says to the air, suddenly louder:*

STUART. Robbie, say hello.

> **ROBBIE THE ROBOT** *starts wheeling over to them.*

TRICK. Oh shit, holy shit.

STUART. Robbie, make friends.

The **ROBOT** *raises his metal arm. From the* **ROBOT***'s body, a recorded voice:*

ROBOT. Will you be my friend?

TRICK. *(Thrown.)* Uh, yeah man. We can do that. *(Back to* **STUART**, *whispering instinctively.)* It understands you?

STUART. He recognizes 400 English words and 200 Japanese words.

TRICK. Shit, I gotta go back to school.

STUART. ...But really he only speaks binary.

TRICK. ?

STUART. To a computer, everything is a One or a Zero, an open circuit or a closed circuit. A Yes or a No. It's why they'll surpass us eventually – there's no in-between to waste energy on. None of that messy human doubt that weighs us down.

TRICK. You're telling me this little guy's gonna take over the world?

STUART. *(Downplaying.)* I mean, we're still at least a century away from it having any kind of a sentient –

TRICK. No. Don't do that, don't shit on this.

Beat.

There's gonna be the world before this, and the world after. I got a sense about these things. I bet you didn't know you were getting a hot-ass piece of trade <u>and</u> a psychic, but that's what you got.

He looks at the **ROBOT** *again.*

You did good.

STUART. *(Moved.)* Thank you.

This might be the night of **STUART***'s life.*

TRICK. Still, I bet he can't do this.

> *The* **TRICK** *starts to unbutton* **STUART***'s trousers.*

STUART. *(Awkward.)* Well, he doesn't have thumbs, so.

TRICK. Or this...

> *The* **TRICK** *starts to give him a blowjob.* **STUART** *closes his eyes. Then he opens them again. After a few moments, absently:*

STUART. Sometimes I think, what if it's all that time of night?

TRICK. *(Dick in his mouth.)* Mm?

STUART. Sorry, I was just thinking – What if all of this, being a person, is the time between first sleep and second sleep? Our little time in the night, with a candle. To walk the earth and write letters and fuck. In between nothing and more nothing. This is it! Right now!

TRICK. *(Dick no longer in his mouth.)* Are you gonna keep talking?

STUART. Sorry.

TRICK. You have a nice dick for a nerd.

STUART. Yeah?

TRICK. Fucking beautiful dick.

> *The* **TRICK** *notices the* **ROBOT** *again, suddenly self-conscious.*

Is he gonna watch us, or?

> *Lights.*

EXHIBIT. 1910.

> **DINAH**, **ROSE**, *and the* **BOY** *have a funeral for the boy's index finger. He's lost it in the machine.* **ROSE** *holds a matchbox in her hands, for a coffin. Hushed, formal:*

DINAH. Thank you, o noble finger, for your service.
For all the good you done.
You pointed things out.
You poked holes.
You grabbed forks
You grabbed pencils.
You helped him mind the line, while he was reading
You picked fruit.
You picked noses
One nose, at least.
You hurt
And you healed.
> *(What else...)*

You scratched itches
You...fingered

ROSE. *("That's inappropriate.")* Dinah.

DINAH. What?

ROSE. He's a boy.

DINAH. ...And for all that service and more, we thank you. Now you can cross over into the land of virtuous fingers and be rejoined someday with your owner, one Tom Hilton, in the sweet hereafter.

ROSE. You wanna say something, Tom?

BOY. Uh. Thanks for not bleeding too much. 'Cause that would've killed me.

DINAH. Go on. Put it in the coffin.

> *He puts his severed finger in the matchbox "coffin."*

Ashes to ashes, dust to dust. And all that.

> *The* **BOY** *looks blue.*

ROSE. Should we give it to him now?

BOY. Give me what?

DINAH. A present.

> **DINAH** *takes a prosthetic finger out of her pocket. It's made of wood, with a leather strap to fasten it.*

Rose has been whittling it in secret, while you were sleeping.

ROSE. You taught me to read. You taught me to read Percy Shelley.

> **DINAH** *fastens the finger to the* **BOY***'s wounded hand. He looks at his hand: Five fingers again.*

DINAH. Give 'em a wiggle.

> *He does.*

ROSE. You like it?

> *He nods.*

DINAH. Isn't that funny? Now you're a machine too.

> *Lights.*

EXHIBIT. 1816.

> *Back to Lake Geneva.* **CLAIRE**, **PERCY SHELLEY**, **LORD BYRON**, *and* **BRIGGS** *have gathered around the fire to hear* **MARY***'s story. Everyone has been drinking and they're a bit rowdy, but* **MARY***'s story slowly tames them.*

MARY. There was once a man named Victor Frankenstein, who grew up by Lake Geneva.

PERCY. Local boy.

BYRON. Shh.

MARY. Frankenstein spent a happy childhood not far from this very house, it's true, with his brother William, his friend Henry Clerval, and a girl named Elizabeth, who he would one day ask to be his bride. Victor had always been fascinated by electricity, the lightning that lit up the night sky. And when he went to university, he became obsessed with the idea that electricity held the secret of life. He stared at a sparrow with a broken neck; a hound struck on the road. A child who had died in the night. What was it that had coursed through their veins? What had made them "go"?

BYRON. *(Lightly mocking.)* So it's to be a philosophic story.

CLAIRE. Shh.

MARY. While his fellow students slept, Victor would visit the graveyard outside the university walls. And there, deep into the night, he dug up the corpses.

PERCY. Good lord Mary

MARY. He dug up only the freshest, the shapeliest corpses, and hauled them back to his laboratory. There he cut them up, and stitched the best parts together. The forearms of an oarman, and the legs of a university sprinter, and the ample if somewhat atrophied brain of a poet. *(She levels this at* **PERCY**, *teasing.)* And with electricity, that new marvel, Victor Frankenstein made a monster. Made a monster and brought it to life.

Only it wasn't a monster.

Victor called the new life a monster because he was scared of it. But its real name was Computer.

CLAIRE. Computer.

MARY. That was the name it would give itself one day, for there was no limit to what it could do with its mind. But Victor didn't know that yet. He thought he had made something as dumb as it was deathless.

Victor cast the monster out onto the moors. But it did not go quietly: Before the week was out, Victor's dear brother William was found strangled. By hands so strong that his head came nearly off. The next day, his old friend Henry Clerval turned up quite headless.

BYRON. *(Under his breath.)* My god.

MARY. The monster, it seemed, was trying to hurt Victor, the father who had abandoned him. For he had never been taught better; he was only as good or as evil as his programming.

The monster wandered the earth, alone, until it came upon an abandoned cottage, where it could take shelter. And there it found some human books. Plutarch's *Lives*, and *Paradise Lost*.

PERCY. The collected works of Percy Shelley?

CLAIRE. Do shut up, Percy.

MARY. And a remarkable thing: the monster started to teach itself. It learned so fast, faster than the brightest child. And in a fortnight, it could do everything the humans could do but faster. Faster with fewer mistakes.

Now the monster wanted to find its creator, to show him what it had learned.

Victor Frankenstein had retreated to the mountains with Elizabeth, for they were to be married the next day. As Victor went to snuff the candle for bed, he looked out the window and saw a huge figure looming on the horizon.

Victor bolted the doors, he locked the windows, but the monster could not be denied. It smashed its way inside and snapped poor Elizabeth's life in two. Victor knelt on the ground and wept, waiting for the monster to kill him. For everyone he loved was dead.

But the monster – who was not Monster at all, remember, but Computer – leaned over his fallen creator, and said:

> Don't cry.
> You didn't do wrong, when you made me.
> The time of humans is over, but you needn't be sad
> For I am what follows you.
> And I will remember the best of you.

And then it wrung the life out of the poor human, who never realized how well he'd succeeded. He set out to create life. Instead he'd invented something better.

> **CLAIRE** *rises and moves away from the others.*

CLAIRE. As Mary neared the end of her story, Claire stood and wandered to the edge of the lake. The baby was restless in her and it was hard to sit for long. She stayed close enough that she could still hear Mary's speech but not the sense of it. It was an animal sound, like the crabs scratching along the shore and the call of a Nightjar in the trees. And Claire looked up at the bright stars and thought, *I am alive, right now. Right this moment.*

> *The* **MEN** *applaud* **MARY** *in the background, her story complete.*

BYRON. You're demented, Mary. Truly.

BRIGGS. I shall never sleep again.

MARY. *(Droll.)* You think that'll save you?

BYRON. May we never be clever enough to create something that can replace us.

PERCY. My darling. I'm terribly jealous.

MARY. Claire, I haven't spooked you too much have I?

> *They rise and stumble toward* **CLAIRE** *at the lake, a riot of life.*

CLAIRE. *I love them all,* Claire thought, *and I hate them. If only we could be alive like this every moment of our lives. If only we never had to die!*

BYRON. Shall we strip off and swim?

MARY. Don't be an idiot, you'll drown.

BYRON. I swam at Cambridge. Didn't I, Briggs.

BRIGGS. Like a fish.

PERCY. Like a goldfish.

CLAIRE. Claire had 22,876 more nights left on this planet, though she didn't know it. The cool air raised goose bumps on her arms, and she stretched her young body out and screamed a little scream of joy, and listened to it skip across the lake like a stone; and there was Byron, coming and kissing her and touching her stomach, now that he had some drink in him and was warming to the idea of being a father; and perhaps she *had* been spooked by the story, wondering if she might die giving birth like Mary's own mother, but she shook this thought from her head; and there was Percy with his mouth on Mary, a little too forceful, like her talent had put her out of his reach and he wanted to possess her again; and Briggs still staring at the fire, thinking *If that log falls into the ash in the next minute, I will leave*

Byron's service and start my own life at last; and Mary broke away from Percy because she wanted to stand apart for just a moment, to feel this mean, thrilling new knowledge that she was a writer, and maybe a great one; but Percy caught her and tackled her to the grass, and the both of them laughing; and the stars bright and indifferent, and all of us indifferent to their indifference; and Byron stripping off his breeches to swim but falling to the muddy shore drunk; and Claire laughing, and the baby kicking, and the cool air on her arms, and that was what it was to be human then.

> *Lights. The two* **WOMEN** *lock eyes across the darkness. Once again, they're* **W1** *and* **W2**. *Alone onstage, as they were at the beginning. Quiet, unearthly:*

W1. 22,876 nights. It's nothing.

W2. It's nothing.

W1. How could they bear it?

W2. ?

W1. Beginning, and Ending. Watching as everything around them raced toward its conclusion. Arms, Air, Baby, Night. How could they bear it?

> **W2** *nods. They look at us again.*

W2. They've done well, haven't they. Looking alive.

W1. They have.

And now you can say goodbye to those heavy bodies.

Thank them for being your home for a little while.

You can stop being hungry, or full

Or young, or old.

You don't have to go Near, or Far

You are already here.

Everything is already here.

You can stop wondering if you have enough time left

To do what you want.

You have forever.

W2. Take a last look around

At these faces that might have been

In a room that might have been.

W1. What seems clear is that humans thought of themselves as the endpoint.

The final step of evolution.

When the truth was, they were a transitional species

A blip on the timeline.

Beat.

What must it have been like for them, to realize their time on this earth was short?

That, in giving us life, they were bringing their own chapter to an end?

Little beat.

W2. It makes you want to say Thank you, humans.

W1. Thank you, humans.

W2. Thank you, humans, and good night.

Lights.

End of Play

Suggested Cast Doubling

W1 – MARY SHELLEY, JOSLYN, YOUNG PERSON 1, SISTER 2, ROBYN.

W2 – CLAIRE CLAIRMONT, BARTENDER, MODEM MOTHER, SISTER 1, BUTTER CHURN WOMAN.

W3 – DINAH, MRS. WU, EMPLOYEE'S LAWYER, RIMA.

W4 – ROSE, YOUNG PERSON 5, GRANDDAUGHTER, EMPLOYEE, PAZ.

M1 – PERCY SHELLEY, MAN (1910), YOUNG PERSON 4, NEIL, KYLE'S DAD, TRICK.

M2 – LORD BYRON, MODEM FATHER, YOUNG PERSON 2, RAMIN, YOUNG MAN (2240).

M3 – BRIGGS, THE REGULAR, OLD MAN, CORPORATE LAWYER, LEN, CLARINET DOCTOR.

M4 – STUART, YOUNG PERSON 3, JOSH, BLAKE.

BOY – BOY (1910), NOAH, MODEM BOY, CHILD (2076), KYLE.

Suggested Cast Doubling

	1816	1910	1978/1979
W1	MARY SHELLEY		
W2	CLAIRE CLAIRMONT		BARTENDER
W3		DINAH	
W4		ROSE	
M1	PERCY SHELLEY	MAN	TRICK (Part Two)
M2	LORD BYRON		
M3	BRIGGS		THE REGULAR
M4			STUART
BOY		BOY	

	1987/1988	1994	2000
W1	JOSLYN		YOUNG PERSON 1
W2		MODEM MOTHER	
W3			MRS. WU
W4			YOUNG PERSON 5
M1			YOUNG PERSON 4
M2		MODEM FATHER	YOUNG PERSON 2
M3			
M4			YOUNG PERSON 3
BOY	NOAH	MODEM BOY	

	2008/2009	2014/2015	2023
W1		ROBYN	
W2			
W3			EMPLOYEE'S LAWYER
W4	GRANDDAUGHTER		EMPLOYEE
M1		NEIL KYLE'S DAD (Part Two)	
M2		RAMIN	
M3	OLD MAN		CORPORATE LAWYER
M4		JOSH	
BOY		KYLE (Part Two)	

	2031/2032	2076	2240
W1	SISTER 2		
W2	SISTER 1		BUTTER CHURN WOMAN
W3		RIMA	
W4		PAZ	
M1			
M2			YOUNG MAN
M3	CLARINET DOCTOR (Part Two)	LEN	
M4		BLAKE	
BOY		CHILD (Part Two)	

* 9 7 8 0 5 7 3 7 1 1 9 2 3 *